PERFECTION
WITHOUT TRYING

RETURN TO YOURSELF

Victor Christian

PERFECTION WITHOUT TRYING...

~

*T*o all the young girls who are thinking about wearing makeup to cover up that already beautiful face. A face that most women would like to have again. The face you were born with, that only water and kisses from your mother should touch. Stand strong, set the trend, and be yourself forever...the real you.

...And for the women who want to return to themselves, it's a simple process and may be challenging at first, so you too stand strong and take the first step of recovery... stop wearing makeup!

You will not regret it. Reward yourself, it will be the best thing mentally and physically. The weight you carry will become lighter and the stress will melt away. Have the courage to live your life as the real you for the rest of your life.

Return to yourself...

TABLE OF CONTENTS

INTRODUCTION

~

First, I want to tell you that I'm not a fan of all the books and commercials on how lotions, creams, masks, powders, and almost all the other products on the market related to the cosmetic industry will help you maintain healthy skin because they don't! Especially if they are made up of synthetics. They are nothing but advertising, persuading you into thinking they do.

The Introduction of Synthetics of any kind thinking they will assimilate into the human body for the betterment of its natural evolution or improvement, is as wrong a thought as the earth changing direction and reversing time.

It's time to change the way women feel about themselves starting with wearing makeup just to please others. It is, without a doubt, the primary reason for premature aging for women and men as well. Even men involved in the news media or movies apply and remove makeup, which also takes a toll on their skin. A lot of them have aged way beyond their years.

I consider myself the modern-day **Pied Piper**, to lead all young girls away from wearing makeup. Living life thinking you need to wear makeup to look your best, is not the direction you want to go.

I know my intentions will be challenged by many but regardless, the truth about wearing makeup day after day will wreak havoc on your skin and you will look older before your time, and some sooner than you think.

I'm just the messenger, the person not afraid to inform you, to tell you the truth about what others think of you wearing makeup. I will not apologize to those who think I'm being a bit harsh, but the process of applying makeup and removing it no matter in the gentlest or vigorous way will cause premature aging.

It's a Fact: For women who already have wrinkles all over their face, foundations of any kind will not fill in the cracks or crevices, on the contrary, it only makes the lines more prevalent, even larger, and we see it, we notice it.

I will admit that there are those with artistic abilities, who can sometimes enhance one's appearance, without distortion, but very few, but that's not the point of this book. Wearing too much makeup and removing it will age your face. The unblemished beautiful first layer of skin will not last long if you start wearing makeup or don't stop.

The best preservation method for the skin on your face is to leave it alone. Let your go-to face, be the natural you.

(Search Damaged Skin from Makeup Use)

Wearing Makeup dates all the way back to 600 B.C., starting with the Egyptians. But I'm not going to explain why, that's what the internet's for. Loads of history on makeup, who first began to wear it, and why.

Of course, it was fashionable for women to wear more conspicuous make-up. mostly influenced today, by Hollywood and all its glamour. Film stars, theater, and exotic dancers, just to name a few. Of course, today, it's blown way out of proportion.

In the late 60's and 70's Hippies began a trend of not wearing makeup. Currently, in Hollywood, it seems the trend is coming back.

Surfer Girls, who are known as natural beauties, let the Sun and Surf sustain a healthy lifestyle and always a beautiful look. My favorite of choice.

There are a lot of sports female athletes who do not wear makeup, at least most of them before, during, or after the game.

The Amish, Quakers, and Mennonites never wear makeup.

Early damage begins when you first apply makeup and the process of removing it. Search online for the words" Young Teens without makeup" and you'll see a slew of pictures showing pictures of girls with bruising around the eyes. That's just the start of unavoidable damage. Yikes!

Some might think that's just a part of wearing makeup and growing up. Well, you will not think that way when the bruising and stretched skin is so bad, that you need to wear makeup to cover all the damage. Thus, the unfortunate cycle begins. The trick is to never start.

I'm confident my message is easy to understand. I'm simply trying to present the facts about aging prematurely. If you read and comprehend the information, you'll remain younger-looking than all your friends. In fact, you could start a trend within your click, your group. It's as simple as this: " You want to stay looking younger your entire life, don't start wearing makeup.

Of course, a huge percentage will exclaim: *"No Way, I'll never stop wearing makeup" or "I've got to wear makeup"*. Yes, you probably do now, if you've started to wear makeup every day. Putting it on before school or shopping, taking it off after you get home, then applying it again, before going out, and then removing it again, and again and again.

First, you'll never match the once-perfect face you owned before wearing makeup. Meaning, that when you first apply makeup and remove it over and over, you've lost the original layer of beautiful skin you were born with. The Natural You will disappear. It's sad, very sad.

It's very noticeable to me when women are out grocery shopping or in the mall somewhere. They might look in my direction but quickly look away, because they have lost the look they once had, and I must say it was preventable, it is no one's fault but their own. More makeup has never meant more beauty.

What's even sadder, is when women go out with their husbands, and apply more makeup over already applied makeup, which only brings out the wrinkles even more.

Did you know that most men prefer their wives to wear makeup before going out? Why? Because they want them to cover the dark circles, bruising, and blemishes caused by the process of wearing makeup in the first place.

I want to persuade the younger generation not to fall into the same pattern. You don't have to, it's not a law, and it's not necessary to have more friends, get good grades, or drive safely. It is not a rite of passage as you get older. It's not a sign of respect to venture into public with makeup on.

In fact, if you never start wearing makeup, you'll remain younger-looking than any of your friends who do wear makeup. It's a proven fact. Anyone who applies makeup and removes it every day will eventually grow older-looking than those who don't. Some might say, *"Oh, I don't care, I want to look older for my new boyfriend."*

"All my friends wear makeup, so I do too." If **you do** start wearing makeup at a young age, you will regret ever starting, because every day you apply the makeup and remove it, no matter the method, you're taking away a layer of youth.

There will be people explaining how they can apply makeup to make you look special, but it is a fact that if you start wearing makeup, you'll begin a process of always wearing makeup to cover the imperfection, the damage you'll cause over the years. In fact, you will look older than you really are, I see it every day.

The one thing I do know, you cannot tread over the skin day after day without pulling, pushing, and stretching the skin. It's a fact that the skin stretches, especially around your eyes, the eyelids {Nasolabial) being the easiest to stretch as well as the skin above the upper lip.

I know you may not like what I have written about something you may have looked forward to doing as a young girl. But, try to absorb as much of this information as possible, and use it as a reference, to help maintain the natural radiance in your skin, staying secure with the face you have.

Look, men and women see a difference in their faces every morning. They might notice puffiness around the eyes, because of too much sodium they ingested in a meal the day before. Drinking and smoking all night long causes a change in appearance. The lack of staying properly hydrated may make the wrinkles in the face more pronounced.

The regimen presented in this book doesn't require creams, lotions, masks, or any cosmetics or other expenses. It's up to you to be consistent with the routine and have patience with the results.

If you have not started wearing makeup and never intend to, well you should be proud of that decision, because it's the only way to not age like many of the women ahead of you. and even those who have been wearing makeup for 20 or more years, can stop and begin the stages of recovery.

"I know I repeat myself, maybe more than a few times, but the great psychologist, Jean Piaget once said, Repeat, Repeat, Repeat. It's the best idea of extreme influence on the mind."

PERFECTION WITHOUT TRYING

~

"Return to yourself"

Victor Christian

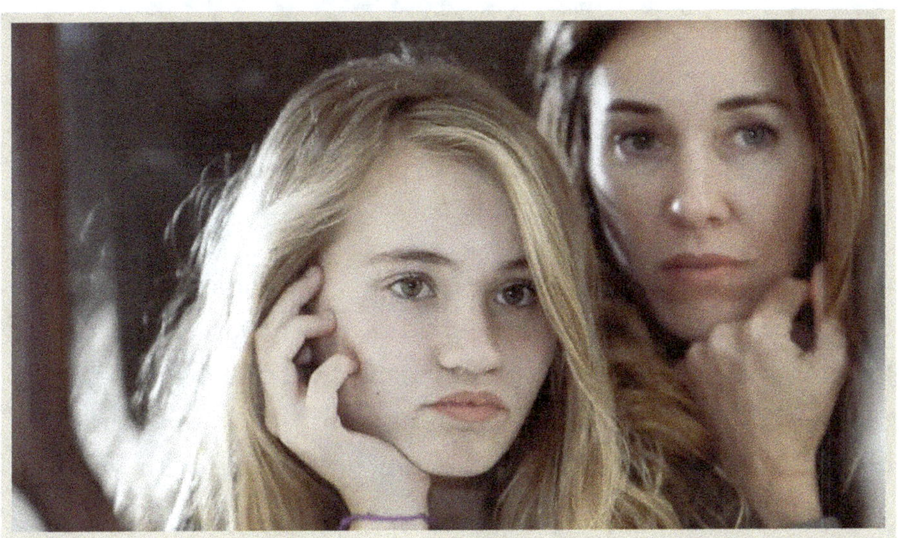

First, I'd like to state the obvious, it's your choice to look like a natural beauty all your life or a worn-out has-been before you're 30. Don't take it from me, just search women with and without makeup, and you may be shocked.

Of course, for young girls, it's an unfortunate transition from an untouched face to when you start wearing makeup. You'll second-guess yourself the first time you apply the makeup and wonder if others approve of the new you. Your boyfriend, best friend, mom, dad, school friends?

In the beginning, don't count on anyone saying *"Wow, your makeup is off the charts"* It may not happen. Unfortunately, you'll continue to change your face day after day, no matter what. It's what everybody does, all your friends and relatives. Really? Do you really have to put on your makeup? I wrote this little book for young girls who might be thinking about wearing makeup for the first time and for those who are already wearing makeup and have been for years. Of course, there'll be never-ending persuasion from siblings, girlfriends, and even mothers when they feel the time is right for you to use makeup. Surprisingly enough, some mothers don't suggest wearing makeup at all and let their daughters decide on their own.

For most young girls, they feel it's a graduation point of life to be recognized as being more mature, and a step towards being a young lady in society with more respect. Yet, I have to say right now, without hesitation, you're turning your back on the everlasting beauty God gave you for your entire life. A face with youthful delicate skin.

A mother's kissable face forever. Yet, most choose to begin applying powders, creams, and coverups that will inevitably wear away their beautiful skin in the rigorous process of removing it day after day.

Of course, every little girl wants to feel more grown up and fit in with their group. Most do not foresee the future of the path they're about to take. The weight placed on their shoulders will be uncomfortable and maybe embarrassing at times, especially when they first start to wear makeup. You'll ask yourself; *"Do I look all right? "Did I put it on correctly? "Why did my boyfriend and family laugh as soon as they saw me in makeup?*

The indecisive task of wearing makeup begins early. Simply put, applying the makeup will involve pushing, rubbing, and spreading makeup, sometimes aggressively, always in a hurry. Thus begins the stretching. This is the truth; I'm not making this up.

Then the worst damage comes from removing it. Over time the resilience in your skin will become weaker and weaker. The elasticity will fade quickly. Eventually, if not sooner, the eyelids will begin to droop, after removing eyeliner and makeup on the eyelids, Yikes! Stretch City! That once untouched virgin skin, the natural smooth skin you were born with will begin to look different, yes, even when you're just beginning. You will find yourself looking closely in the mirror, after the first task of removing it.

Why let anyone make your choices involving a long process of unnecessary stressful labor trying to enhance your natural beauty when it's already with you? Why not start the trend of not wearing makeup and continue being the real you? Be the one whom your friends want, *"to be like"*. It's without a doubt in my mind, that your boyfriend will love it and be proud to be with you.

I'm here to tell you, that if you choose to let the TV Commercials and Hollywood guide the use of makeup and cosmetics, it will end up destroying your skin and the natural beauty you were born with.

All the young girls and women in the commercials are wearing tons of makeup and or airbrushed without a doubt, and you know this. Why? It's a way of selling their products and younger people want to *be like* the people they see in the commercials. You begin to succumb to the subliminal messages. The hype.

If you could only see those young girls and women in those commercials without their makeup, and maybe you have, it should be a warning to you and your friends.

There's not a single woman in Hollywood or elsewhere for that matter, who has been wearing makeup for a long time, that does not have brownish stains and bruising caused by applying makeup and more so by the task of removal.

Some might say, it's simply a part of wearing makeup. So, get ready for the transformation of your once beautiful face, to put it bluntly, to a worn-out look. Of course, I think there is no gentle way to remove lots of makeup on delicate skin. It's the worst process you'll experience and does not and will not prolong beauty.

Of course, peer pressure will not set you free. It will be a struggle for most. But you can help change the way women look and feel about themselves. You can begin the trend of not wearing makeup and being just yourself. Why place this type of worry on yourself, when you don't have to?

Young girls simply have no aging around their forehead, eyes, cheeks, and neck. The whites of their eyes are bright, and their lips are smooth with a pinkish hue. I'm here to tell you, right now in this book, you can keep this and maintain this natural beauty longer than most if you simply don't start wearing makeup.

As a man who's still startled when I meet or happen to be in the same room as a beautiful woman wearing no makeup. I call them "Natural Beauties ", sometimes "Island Beauties" I can't help staring. Just last night while shopping at WF a young lady caught my eye. A young natural beauty. Lightly tanned, thick eyebrows, and absolutely no makeup. Wow! She stood out among all the other women wearing makeup.

Some might say, it's a diamond in the ruff. Why can't women forget about society and commercials that do nothing but try and persuade you to purchase their products?

We all know, it's a billion-dollar industry, but only good for fake beauty. In the past, "Animal Testing" was part of cosmetic production.

Cruelty to animals. Testing out the chemical-filled products. Yes, cosmetics are still processed and manufactured with synthetic chemicals, and some contain carcinogens.

Please note: You will not ever need any of these products if you never touch your face with makeup to begin with. Isn't that a wonderful feeling? Not to have the worry of makeup in your life? Trust me, the shiny, greasy, powdery face is not a good look on anyone, and we see it all day long. Women on the news, variety shows, game shows. Of course, I comment to myself every time I see a *"too much makeup girl"*

Do older women think that men would rather see them with a few wrinkles or a face with a few wrinkles covered up with powders or creamy foundation coverups, that do nothing but enhance the appearance of wrinkles, making them look like cracks in a desert landscape? For those women who do this, it looks distracting, horrible, and more noticeable. Trust me on this, it's what everyone sees. Let the truth be known. It's not attractive.

JUST THE FACTS:

The removal of makeup every night, scraping, pulling, and rubbing is the foremost way of damaging your skin. All those who do show evidence of skin damage early in life, results in premature aging. It is inevitable.

Consequences for life: End it now, before you're trapped, always feeling the need to wear makeup before being seen in public.

But wait, there's more... It is reversible, but it will take a strong-willed person to follow a strict recovery regimen. To include nutrition, hydration, and exercise to return to themselves. No Surgery is needed.

Sadly, we all see some turn to Plastic Surgery, which looks downright comical, and to make things worse, they wear makeup over their plastic surgery to hide the surgical scars.

In the end, some even become recluses. Please, ladies, don't become victims of plastic surgery. Have faith in yourselves stop wearing makeup, get on a nutritional diet, and complete the recovery.

If you cut yourself and the wound heals on its own, that should tell you that you can recover from dark circles and bruised skin on your face. You can recover from the damage.

Oh, and BTW, If you think others can't tell you have had Plastic Surgery, think again. That's like not noticing when a man is wearing a hairpiece, right?

Such a beautiful face, but already shows bruising around the eyes from a regimen of makeup removal.

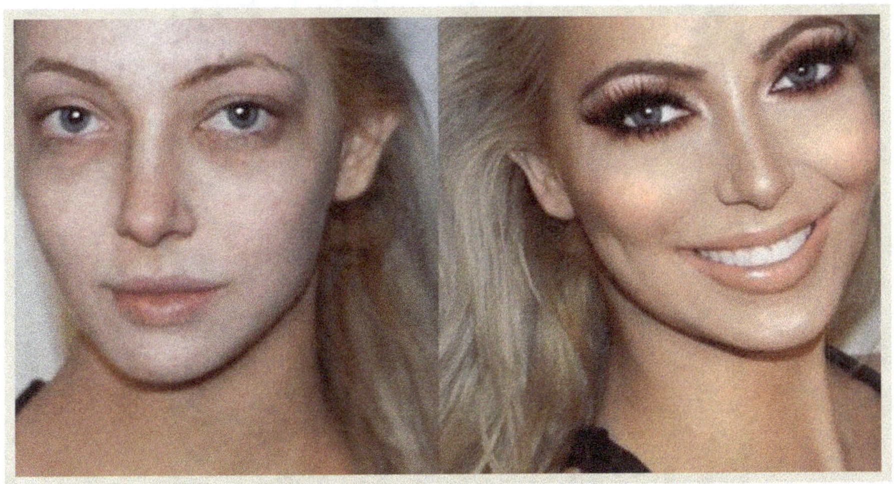

So, ask yourself, do I want to start wearing makeup or should I follow the recovery regimen to maintain my natural beauty for the rest of my life?

If you do follow my regimen, you will look as pretty as can be, your entire life, a Natural Beauty and if you decide to wear makeup as your go-to-fake-face, you'll eventually look worse than you can ever imagine when you get older, that's inevitable. Young girls who start wearing makeup may end up using it for the rest of their lives, as I've explained already. That is the truth.

Most Natural Beautiful Women all over the world are most admired for their healthy radiant skin, with no signs of ever wearing makeup. No matter who they are, they are easy to recognize all through the years of their life. Be confident in yourself and the way you appear to others. Especially at your high school reunions.

I would never attempt to create a face prettier than the woman in the picture below.

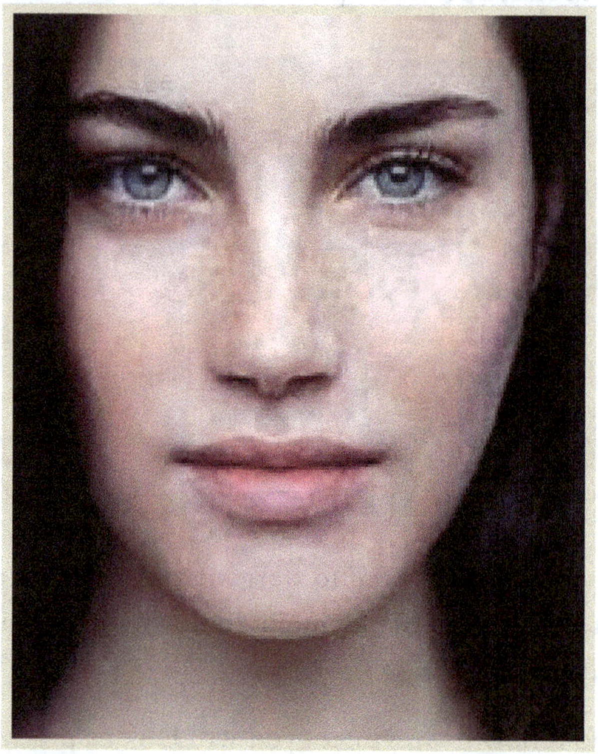

Most women are not talented enough to apply makeup better than the face you're born with, leaving a natural appearance. On the contrary, most bombard their face with tons of makeup, thinking the more the better. Some look clownish... end up looking older than they are.

The unskilled will put on and take off several times a night or day, while never being satisfied with the last attempt.

Eventually, over the years, you'll be one of those, who will scream in the mirror, ***"Oh, I need to put on my makeup, I look terrible"*** So if you begin wearing makeup, even if you don't need it, and if you're wearing too much makeup, you're heading down a path, that will eventually destroy, what once was your natural youthful beauty, which is envious of all who have gone before you.

I wish I could shout out on a stage in front of thousands of Females. ***"You don't need to wear makeup."***

Furthermore, almost every young woman follows the norm of wearing makeup. Most hurry in the morning, rushing to school or work, looking like a Broadway musical character, a clown, or just plain silly, sometimes leaving chunks of mascara on their eyelashes, totally unaware. Some paint the sides of their cheeks, forehead, and around their eyes, not knowing it's a huge dark mask seen by everyone.

Ease the Frustration and unnecessary worry...

Would it not be more refreshing to start the day with a shower, washing your hair, and maybe just glossing your lips? for the rest of your life? Not ever worrying about make-up. What a frustrating hassle, expense, and needless worry you place on yourself.

I say that because Men don't. They are, who they are, and that's all you get. Like it or not. They don't put a Mask on, and then take it off at night. Men remain easily recognizable throughout their lives. It is a known fact that men age better than women. Ever wonder why?

I'm confident I've written words to live by, so you can remain a Natural Beauty the rest of your life, never having to hide the real you behind a mask or fake this or fake that. In only 3 Words, "Don't Wear Makeup."

I hope you'll keep this book as a good reference, so you can teach others. The Fountain of Youth has always been with you..., your time and devotion are all you need.

If you've been wearing makeup for some time now.... have the courage to just stop...be proud of who you are....

Return to yourself...

Early in life, as a young boy, I sometimes watched my mother perform a nightly routine on her face while trying to get some mom time before going to bed.

Like most women, she wore makeup, and to remove it, she would spread lotion all over her face, then with a soft cloth, remove the lotion and makeup along with it. Night after night for years. It was her regimen.

My Mother was a Natural Beauty, and I was always curious, as to why such an already pretty woman, would want to apply Makeup.

Because it's what women did.

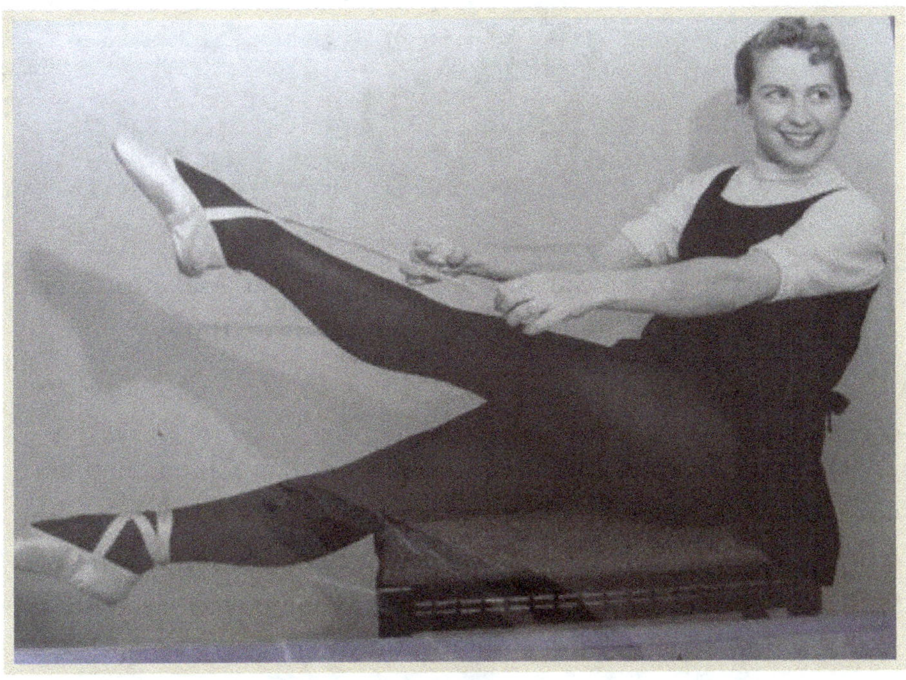

What do Men Want?

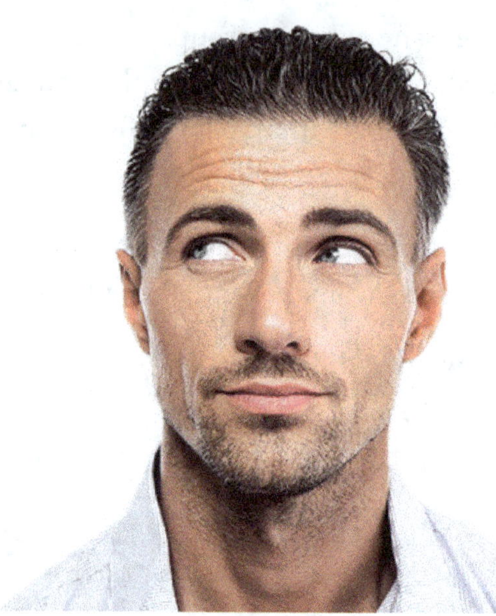

Men want to set the record straight about Makeup, Breast Enhancement, and Fake anything and everything.

Real Men don't approve!

Whether in America, Italy, Greece, France, or China, men have always been attracted to Women, with naturally flowing healthy hair, natural sun-touched skin, and bright gleaming smile. A woman with a Scent all their own. These are the Women who stand out no matter where they are, the all-natural woman with a scent they've owned since childhood.

A huge turn-on for men, but when it comes to makeup, I've never known any guy, who likes to be with a young girl or woman, only to have the makeup rub off her and onto them. It was a knee-slapping joke among teenage boys growing up. Heavy makeup to almost every man I know, is a huge turnoff.

Oh, some may not admit it, but when a natural beauty enters the room, weaving her way through, all eyes are on her. Fortunately for me, I see these women from time to time, and some I've approached just to tell them how beautiful they are without wearing makeup.

There's an easy way to become, what I call a Natural Beauty... very sheik. Trust me on this... like my friend Barbie below. She is and will always be a Natural Beauty.

She turned 30 when this picture was taken.

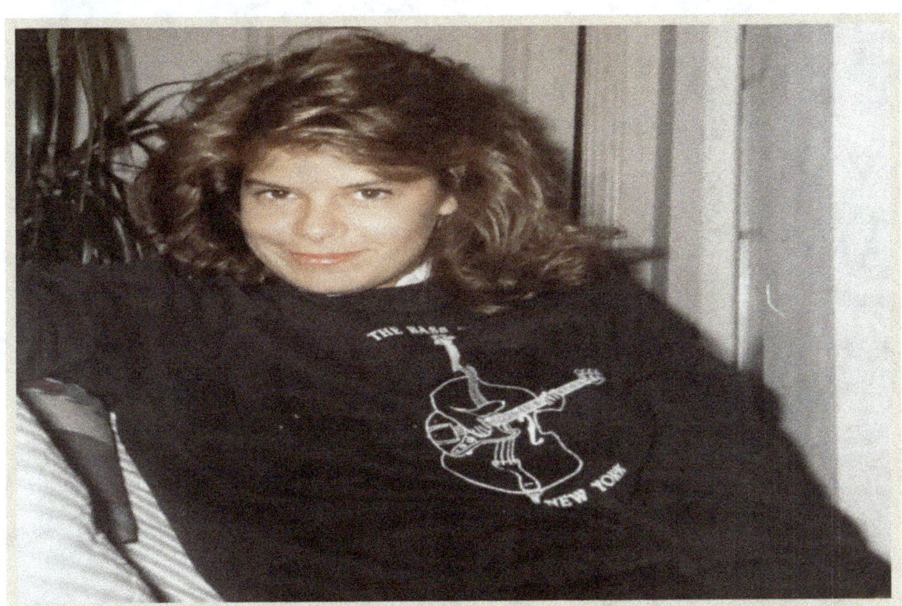

Of course, women of color should never ever have to apply makeup. Their features are all so pronounced that makeup would only distort their natural appearance. They are Perfection Without Trying"

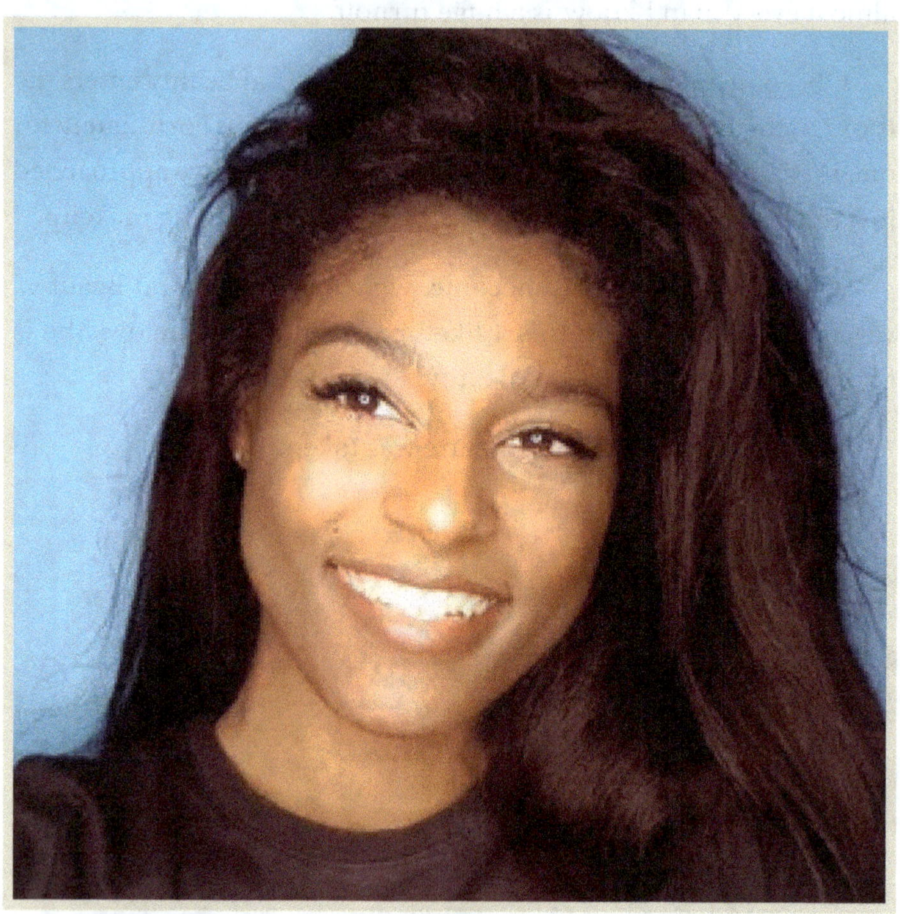

CHAPTER 1

Cosmetics

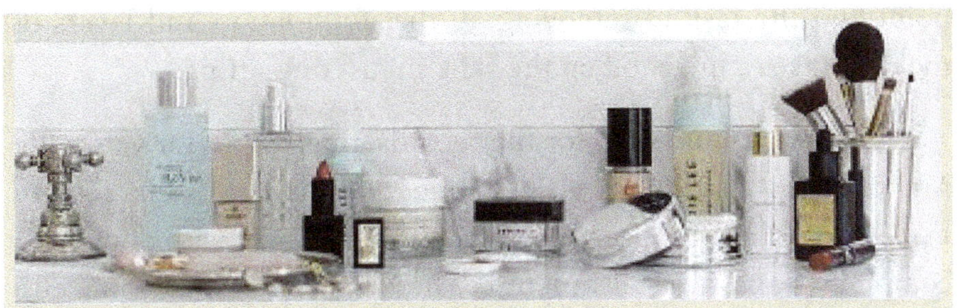

I'm not a fan of Cosmetics. I've never been turned on by women who wear makeup, never have, and never will be. To me, it does not make sense for an already beautiful woman to cover, distort, or misshape their face with makeup. Most young girls and women, apply way too much makeup to begin with.

Here's the deal, to take off all that makeup takes a huge toll on your skin. It doesn't melt off, you must rub it off with cosmetic cotton wipes, or soft light rags of some sort. It's not an easy task. To do this several times a day, YIKES! Stretch City!!! Can you imagine what a Clown goes through or a Broadway Dancer? Or You?

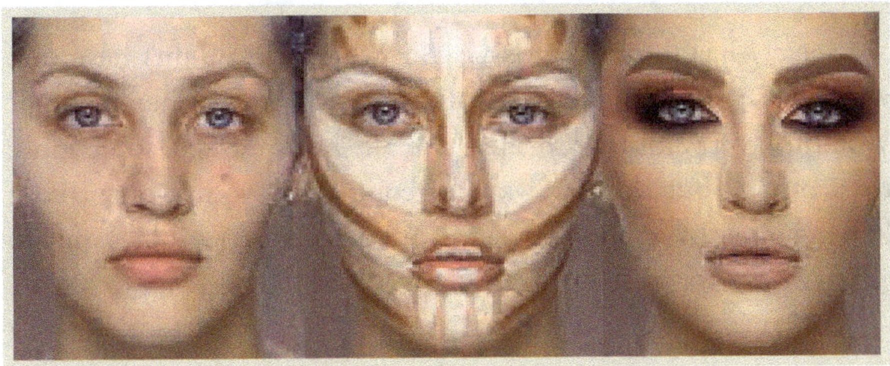

The Method of Contouring the face surfaced when bruising, discoloration started appearing on the face more and more over the years. Makeup artists felt it was a must, for a better balance of the makeup to be applied. Maybe a good foundation for a Clown or Entertainer, but still, whatever you put on, must come off at some point and the task of removing all that foundation and layers of makeup takes a huge toll on the skin, in just one sitting.

However, I must state for the records, that I'm all for Cosmetic Makeup for those who need to correct or enhance a facial feature because of injury, or disease or are simply not born with enough to complete the basic facial structure. There are a lot of skilled makeup artists available to help train you to apply makeup to an optimum level. Please reach out for their help.

My primary reason for this book is to try persuading young girls to never start wearing makeup. Why? You don't need it. You have all the magnificent features most older women want. If you start wearing makeup, you will be like most women, who continue to use it every day to cover up the damage they inflicted over the years.

In my lifetime, I've noticed women age as they get older and I know it hurts them deep inside, to the point of them trying anything and everything to look younger. It's a huge concern for them and doesn't need to be.

Society has forced that issue. But what if you didn't have that worry, and your daughter didn't have that worry in her lifetime? Wouldn't you want that for her? We all show our age, some more than others, but do you want to compound your worry about looking older by applying makeup on the existing wrinkles only to make them more pronounced? Of course not, but most don't have the courage to let go.

Do you want to continue to stretch the skin when you get older removing makeup, still, more and more?

This Scandinavian woman on the next page, like most girls when they were young, wore makeup, but fortunately, as you can see, she's a beautiful woman of 74 living her life without a gorilla on her back, badgering her to put her makeup on.

She returned to herself.

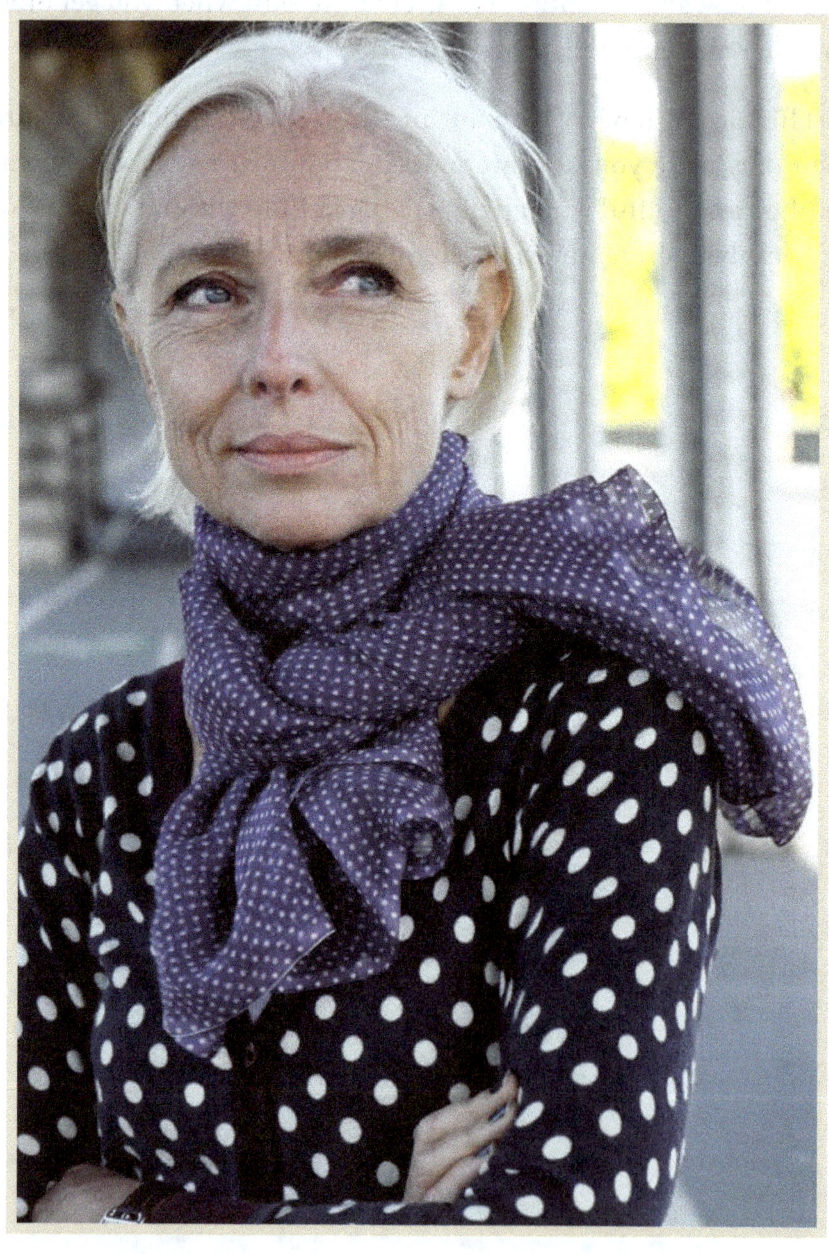

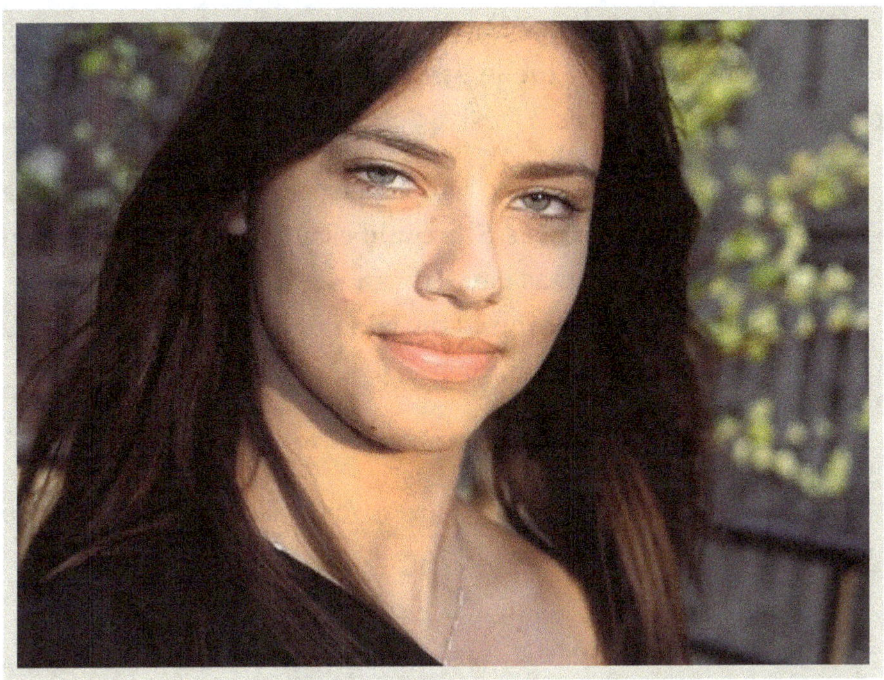

I remember talking with Tristan, a young attractive waitress, one evening in Dallas. As she was explaining her lifelong plans, I was busy noticing the Circus style makeup she was wearing, almost comical, and unaware to her, that it was not very becoming. She had so much makeup on, I could smell it. I thought to myself, here sits a beautiful woman under all that cover-up. Our conversation ended, and she left me wondering.

About an hour later, a young lady walked by on the way out the door, touched my shoulder, and told me "Goodbye, hope to see you again, when you're back in town". "Again? I asked, gently guiding her down to sit... *we haven't met yet*" *"Of course, we have, about an hour ago."*

Wow! It was Tristan...with her makeup completely removed. I was astonished, to say the least. I could see a slight area of dark bruising around her eyes. Yikes!

She was wearing a black motorcycle jacket...and faded blue jeans with holes in the knees. She could easily be taken for a Calvin Klein model. It was clear as day; Tristan was one of those naturally beautiful women, at last, I found my Natural Island Beauty to place in my book. The perfect example.

Tristan, why would you ever want to cover up this beautiful face?

I hope I persuaded her not to ever wear makeup again and she returned to herself. A Natural Beauty, Perfection without trying...

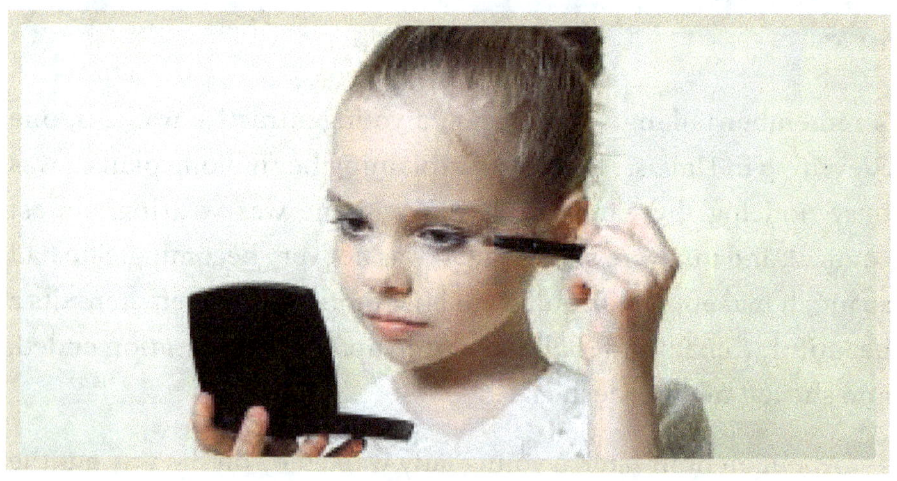

Unfortunately, soon enough, the process begins, and the image in a young girl's mind is wanting to look older and prettier. When she applied makeup for the first time., The first layer of her beautiful skin will inevitably begin to slowly disappear. Just that quick, and she will continue. In that instance, she will let go of the one thing she could have owned forever. To me, that's sad.

I know, I know, it's not all that bad, but I say, yes, it is. I'm hoping to change how young women feel about this stage of their young lives and maybe they'll begin to realize it's not worth all the fuss. I whole heartly feel the process most young girls and women are using in their daily regimens is and will continue wearing out their skin prematurely.

I'm confident the information you will read, will help prevent that from happening and beautiful young girls mature into beautiful women for the rest of their lives.

I have to say, without a doubt in my mind, this is the most critical mistake young women especially teens make. Why would you want to cover up your beautiful skin, smothering, and clogging all your pores? Doing nothing to your skin but making it worse from the start.

Don't you realize that the women ahead of you, the women older than you, wish they had what you have not yet destroyed?

If you are one of those young girls who think you want to look older and prettier by wearing makeup. Well, I have to say, you are wrong. But what comes along with wearing makeup at a young age is more and you may not be ready for it, even if you think so.

Look, most women are always trying to look prettier every time they use makeup. However, each day of applying and removing makeup takes them further away from their goal. But if they continue, no matter what the consequences are. It's too late, they'll never go anywhere without makeup, and they become a victim of the norm, and not really living who they've always been. The real you.

It's a fact that a constant bombardment on the surface of your skin only gets worse, with repeated sessions, AND that's what it will become, sessions sitting in front of a mirror, taking up time in your life, and for what?

But wait, the first big step in recovery is to STOP WEARING MAKEUP. Follow the regimen I've written out and let it become part of your diet for the rest of your life. It's all up to you. You first must stop inflicting damage and begin a natural way of healing.

First, Stop wearing makeup, it is then you begin the process of working for the preservation of your skin's youthful radiance, day after day. If you don't, then, soon your face will need makeup to cover up the inconsistencies, the yellowish-brown bruised skin around your eyes, forehead, and cheeks. You will notice the premature sagging skin under your neck, cheeks, around your mouth, and eyes, as well as other areas you never expected to happen so soon.

I'm just glad I'm writing this to let you know. Most men will not say anything or bring it to your attention.

But let me say this, on occasion, I will see these women without any makeup, and without a doubt, they look worn out. The years of wearing makeup had taken a toll on their natural beauty. Their youth was lost, yet they were still young. Without their makeup, they never looked me in the eye, and usually turned away, eventually rushing to the bathroom or vanity to begin putting on a face, as they called it. So, I ask you, do you want that kind of stress in your life? Hiding until you put your face on? That sounds so ridiculous to even say.

Once young women start wearing makeup, some don't feel attractive without it. I can recall several women in my life, who wore the whole package. Meaning the works, starting with foundation, to eyeliner, mascara, lipstick, blush, and gaudy makeup over the eyes. Nothing that as a man, thought was attractive.

On the other hand, I would sometimes see a few young women without their game face on, ones that had not ventured into wearing makeup for long periods of their lives. Being a huge fan of Natural Beautiful women, I would tell them, how pretty they were and would exclaim, *"Please, when you're with me, never wear makeup"*, and *"You're so beautiful without it"*

Of course, most would blush, because they knew how genuine I sounded in making the statement. Some even got tears in their eyes. To me, it was like gazing into the past, when I didn't even know them, I was seeing how they looked as a very young girl. I even put some to the test. I asked them to put nothing on their face. Some would say, *"I need at least lip gloss"* Then we would go shopping or out to dinner.

Soon with all the compliments, and flirtatious innuendos, I eventually turned them around from looking totally fake to an all-natural beauty with less stress in their life about their appearance at home and in public.

Why are women hiding behind a naturally beautiful face? I hope to change that, and yes, it's possible to reverse the aged look once your mask is off for good. Like anything with our body, it can heal itself. I will teach you how and you'll *return to yourself.*

No more worry or frustration and doubt that you look your best. You've returned to the beauty you've always had with you. Live by your own rules. Stop the hair dye and stop using the Cosmetics with harmful chemicals on your face. Start the natural healing recovery. Have confidence in yourself, and let your self-esteem return for good.

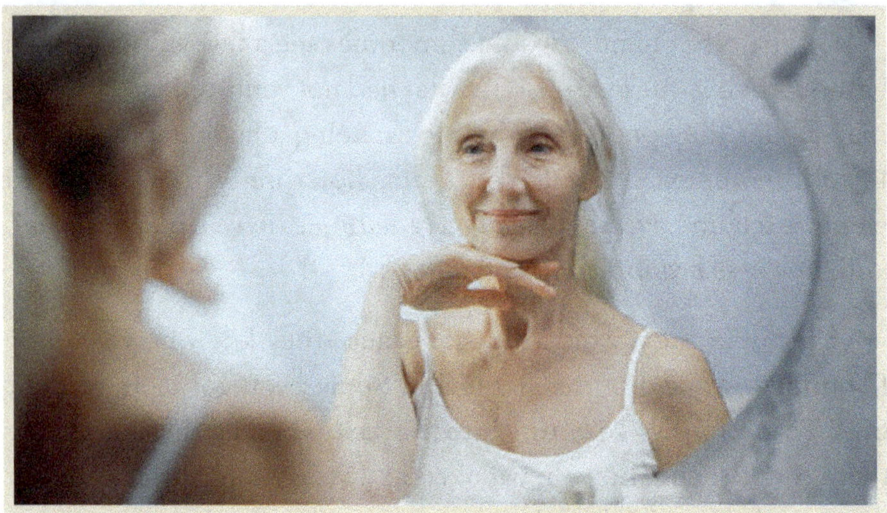

CHAPTER 2

~

Start with Water, End with Water...

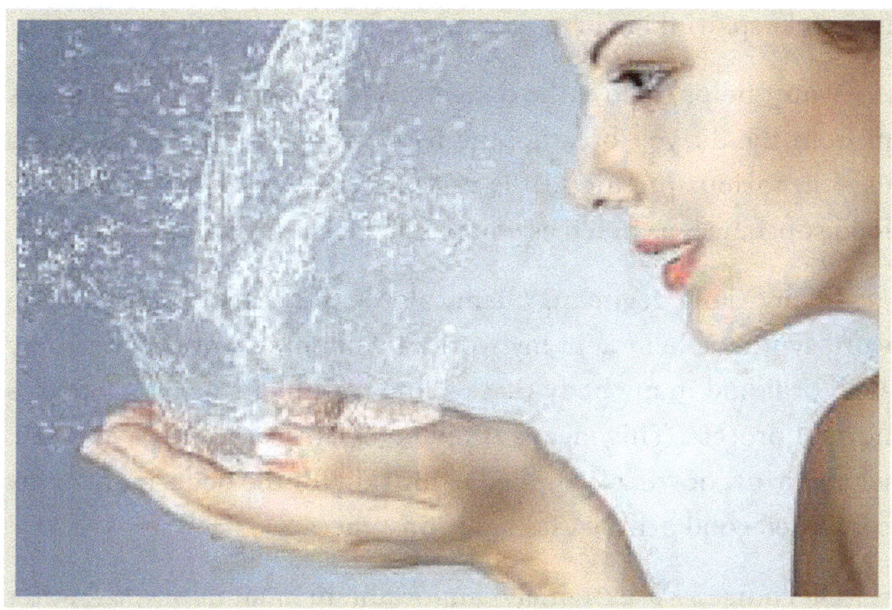

I place the importance of Water at the top of the list. Water regulates your body temperature when it's cold or hot outside. The body needs a regular quantity, and the proper volume to function properly your entire life, throughout the different seasons of the year. If you don't drink enough water every day, all through the day, you will not succeed in your quest to maintain the best skin possible.

That's a scientific fact to maintain beautiful skin throughout your life. All living things on this planet rely on adequate amounts of water.

Your body is made up mostly of water. Approximately 85% of your brain, 80% of your blood, and 70% of your muscles are water. Every cell in your body needs water to live. When you drink water, think of it as the most important substance you're letting flow down your throat into your stomach. Your body will know what to do with it...just keep drinking it.

Water helps remove the dangerous toxins that your body takes in from the air you breathe, the food you eat, and the chemicals used in various products. It is very important to avoid non-whole food substances as much as you possibly can throughout your life.

In my daily regimen, chemicals do not exist, nor does the word synthetic belong in my world. I will not use or consume any solid or liquid in my body that will not assimilate using my body's normal process. This means if my body can't use what I've eaten, what I drink, or what is applied to my skin for the betterment of my continued good health... I do not consume.

Of course, it's extremely important to maintain your water consumption during the summer months, as well as the winter months. If you are a person who sweats a lot, you will need to replace your electrolytes more often than you probably think. Replacing electrolytes in the body, no matter what age, is extremely important, no matter what time of year or location on Earth.

As already mentioned, the body is made up primarily of water, so the balance of water is mandatory.

You can go online to **review Electrolyte and Trace Mineral Replacement** to educate yourself further. I always prefer liquid supplements as they will absorb and assimilate faster than pills or capsules. The ones I use do not contain sugars, fillers, or other unhealthy additives.

Confusing to me, but some might find Water hard to drink unless they're thirsty or just can't stand the taste of water. Oddly enough a huge percentage of people are this way. Unfortunately, this is a huge, majestic size mistake to your health, but it is very easy to fix....one just needs to train or insist they drink more water.

Now, do you personally need to consume 8 /8 oz? glasses of water a day? Maybe not, I believe it all depends on the size of the person you are and your physical stature. Keep in mind, that 8oz. is only 1 measuring cup full. So, drinking that much is not a lot of water...so spread out drinking a cup of water throughout the day.

Here's a good daily regimen to follow upon awakening. Once in the morning (16oz.) 2-cups, then a cup mid-morning (8oz), lunchtime(8-16oz), midafternoon(8oz.), workout period (should be at least 16oz.), and evening. (8oz.)

Please note: whenever you take the time to drink water, announce a -Message to the Brain- in your thought process. See the message and repeat the message. This will train your brain to be aware of the need for water. So, when you are just about to drink your water, say this aloud or silently, it's the thought process and message to the brain that will count. > "The pure clean water I'm drinking is the best thing for my Brain and Body throughout my life." That's your message to the brain. If you don't send the message to the brain, at least I hope you taken note of the message here.

What kind of Water is best to drink? There are reports available to read online, that will tell you. Most all the body's ailments link back to the body not having enough natural Trace Mineral consumption. That's probably because we all drink bottled water. Some water bottling companies are putting minerals back into the water.

Simply read to make sure your favorite bottled water has minerals. If not, there is a simple fix. You can purchase a liquid "Trace Mineral" supplement by adding it to your water consumption. I've found it to be extremely beneficial to my muscles, tendons, ligaments, and bones, just to mention a few. A noticeable difference indeed. You can read more about adding minerals to your water online.

Very important – Your Brain Needs water to function at its best. Always be aware your body sends and receives signals from your brain throughout the day, constantly communicating the only way it can. It's a scientific fact that the brain needs an adequate water supply to send those signals to every part of the body. It's the way it keeps the body functioning in a healthy state. The only problem is, when we're young, we ignore this kind of communication. But, when we get older, every twitch, itch, pain, dizziness, and strain can send us to the brink of acting like a hypochondriac.

Water can be a quick fixer for a lot of funny little feelings here and there. I know this for a fact if you don't drink enough water... towards the end of the day, you may feel a slight headache in the temple area, or your eyes will itch a little. Your skin will appear dry more often, than not and You may even have crappie skin. Easy to fix... Drink more water!

Water can help with Dilution Here's something to remember... after you've eaten that big bag of Potato Chips, a Crispy Crème Doughnut, Chinese food, or a Barbeque Sandwich...try drinking a glass or two of water. Drinking Water will always help dilute everything you eat and lend a hand to your digestive system, all the while keeping you hydrated and maintaining your temperature. You can do this before a meal or after. Doing it before will help control how much you eat.

Please note: You may notice puffiness the next day by eating food with too much sodium/salt in the food. Water will help with dilution, without a doubt.

Water and Sweat It's your body's Natural Cleanser...one of the most important amazing processes of our body. It is your body's exhaust system, a natural way of cleansing from the inside out. We all know, our skin is the largest organ of the body, or some would say on the body or covering the body. So, everywhere you have Skin, you have tiny pores. The body uses a cleansing process where it pushes out dirt, debris, skin dust, leftover lotions, oils, and anything else your skin encounters. Very important for healthy skin throughout your life.

Just think about it for a moment. It's the natural process of your body to sweat or perspire. Otherwise, the pores keep collecting waste, clogging up the exhaust system, which does nothing but wreak havoc on your skin's appearance throughout your life, especially your teenage years. Plus, if impurities can't be eliminated, they usually find their way through the surface of your skin, most commonly on your face, the back of your arms, your chest, and most likely your back. Yes, pimples and or Acne can appear during your teenage, young adulthood, and even into the adult stages of your life.

Something to note to yourself after reading the paragraphs above: If I have pimples now, why do I want to cover them up with makeup, creams, and other oils that are advertised to help? Shouldn't I keep the exhaust system working at 100% to cut down on the number of pimples I have? If I eat a bag of potato chips, peanuts, or chocolate, should I drink a lot of water during and afterward to help my body process eliminating the oils and salt? Yes, you should.

Please note: It is a documented fact that when Chocolate and Nuts are consumed, the body will push the waste/debris to the surface faster than any junk you may consume.

One thing you may not know is if you are using a paste or wax deodorant, YIKES! You're shutting the door and placing a deadlock on your exhaust system. Always use a clean healthy liquid deodorant. Never use cream or wax.

If you have been using wax or paste deodorant, simply stop and use nothing for a couple of days, keep yourself hydrated, exercise vigorously, and or hit the sauna for a couple of sessions so your body sweats the impurities out from the body. The extra water consumption will help clean out your pores. Then if you need to, start using a liquid for the rest of your life. Never, ever clog your armpits.

Of course, after doing this, as we've talked about before, the body also eliminates electrolytes...which you'll need to replace soon after. It's like your car has water but no anti-freeze. Remember how to sweat or perspire? Simply by exercising or in a dry sauna. Both are the best way to help clean out your pores. Did you know hitting the dry sauna is equal to a workout/exercise? Yep, so along with a regimen of exercise, use a dry sauna too. *" start with Water and End with Water..."*

Men and Women can both benefit by splashing cold water on the face as many times a day as possible.

Moisture is your friend. The cold water helps to tighten and close the pores. Splashing ice-cold water after cleansing the face before bed is very beneficial, especially for the pores around the nose.

Start with water, end with water...

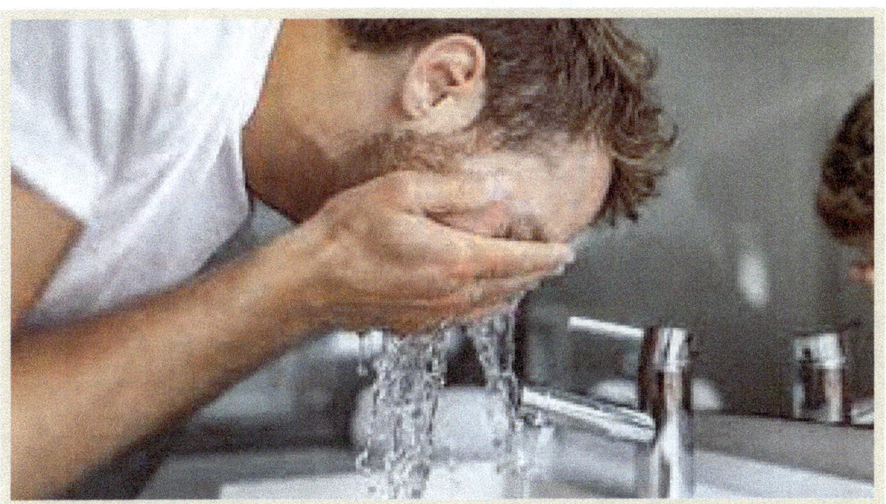

CHAPTER 3

~

Feeding our Mind and Body

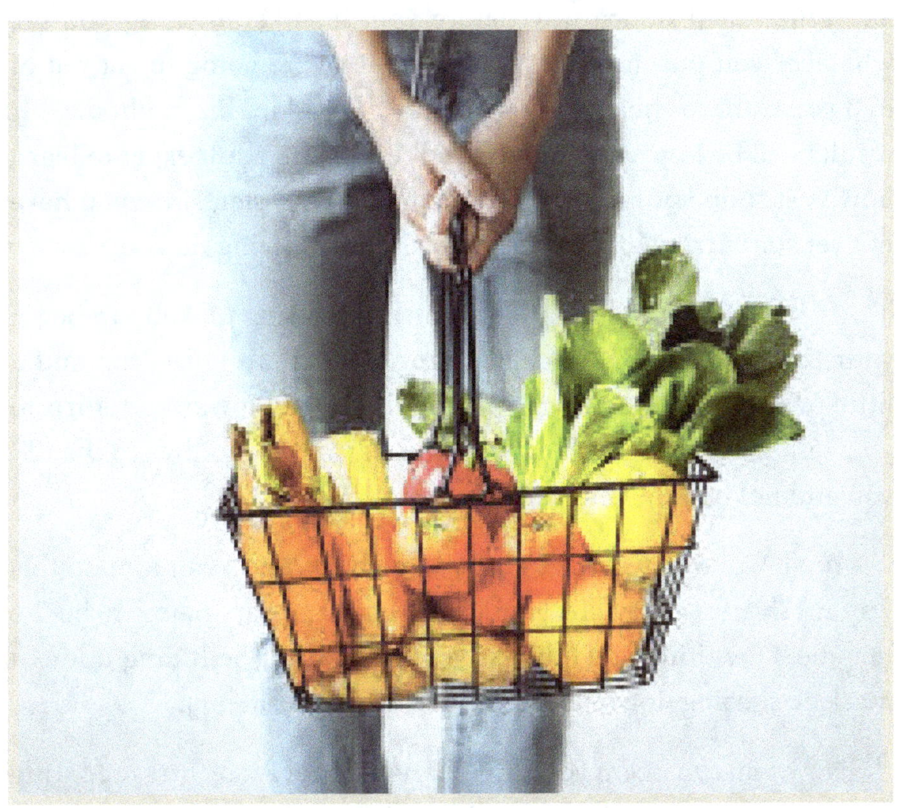

As we all know, starting a new food regimen can prove to be more challenging than climbing to the top of Mt. Everest, for at least some... But the good news is, simply follow my directions and once you get a little over the top...changes will already be apparent. Friends and strangers will begin to take notice of your appearance.

You'll feel the changes in your mood, confidence, and well-being. You'll feel eager to share your experience with others AND...it will not matter what age you are. Changes will take place, I promise you. Be the one to lead by example.

It's very simple, if you follow this regimen, no matter if you're a male or female, young or mature adult, you will achieve changes, and others will notice way before you. It's like anything you do, whatever you put into a project, is what you're going to get out of it. If you want to cheat and just dabble around in this method, your results will be less noticeable. If you're a young adult eager to learn how to sustain your natural beauty, it will be easier, since you have not yet started any bad habits or methods involving makeup.

If you're a little older and are currently using makeup to begin your day, it will be more challenging. The climb to the top and a little over the mountain will be a path directly toward a return to yourself. Once you get there, you will have said goodbye to the old you and hello to the real you.

You'll wonder, wow, I'm glad I came back, and I can remain this way, for the rest of my life. I am what I am…and very happy to be the real me. One thing you'll like is you'll no longer be hiding under a mask or chasing down fake temporary enhancements.

Now, you can begin your life-changing process by first preparing your Food Inventory. I'm not going to list the foods you can eat…as there's plenty of information on the web that will help. However, I will tell you the foods that need to be limited and those are Foods with Sugar, Sodas being the Number 1 on my list to cut out of your life completely. There's way too much sugar in just one can.

Without getting into a long-drawn-out editorial about Sugar Foods, let's just say, you'll have to limit those foods, by making them your treats! This means that occasionally, you can treat yourself to a good whole-food type dessert. I used to be the Poster Boy for Sweets, it is my Kryptonite, but I did succeed in cutting out a lot of sugar in my diet. I did not say all of it, just most of it. I'll be the first to admit the challenge it can be. Just the other day, I was in Whole Foods Market, and as I was walking near their *"Mecca of Sweets Counter"*, the *"OZ of Confections"*, the baker asked, *"Can I help you, sir?"* I responded, *"No thank you, I'm just saying hello to some old friends."* It was very hard to give up such delectable delights, but it is possible. You just must remember my message to the brain, {MTTB} ***"It only tastes good when going over my palate, it does nothing to enhance the health of my body and brain."***

For the last 40 years, I've not swayed too far from my diet, which I've learned was a good way of life for me. My *"diet"* was well established, early on soon after I learned the foods that worked well with my metabolism.

Meaning, that I began selecting among the many fresh foods available from such categories as fish, meats, veggies, and fruits. Then, once I was satisfied with the intake, the output, and the results I put my menu in stone. I admit this takes time and effort on your part. In turn, this made shopping very easy and sometimes fun since it involved trips to the local WF Market.

Placing my "diet" on the top shelf for so many years became second nature to me, a method that my family simultaneously made part of their lives. In doing so, there were fewer, if any, trips to the doctor's office, and not one family relative has ever been hospitalized for an illness, ever.

I must mention that this began with the appreciation of the abundance of food available to all of us, here in America. I began shopping for what I needed for the next couple of days, not a week. This helped with spoilage and needless waste of food. This method along with my preparation of the food I purchased began to help me enjoy the taste and nutrition it provided. I began to enjoy the food I cooked, better than eating out so much.

Before creating your life's menu, realize that you will need to avoid most food products in a box, a can, or for sure, plastic bottles... since most, without a doubt, are manufactured with ingredients that ONLY provide a long shelf life. The people who provide such products do not care about anything you eat, just how long their products can stay on the shelf without spoilage. Therefore, they must put all the artificial ingredients in whatever they prepare. This is where you'll need to use another {MTTB} Message to the Brain. Will my body benefit from the food I'm about to purchase?

Don't make this stressful, just try to be consistent in making the transition from stored food to fresh usable foods. This means whatever you purchase today will need to be prepared and eaten soon or it will spoil. Put on paper your menu for at least 2-3 days, then at the market, shop for the items on your menu. Select and purchase only what you can prepare and eat for a couple of days at a time.

Restaurants do it, and so can you. Your meals will be so much tastier and healthier. If you struggle with cooking, learn. It will be well worth it for you and your family. I'm as guilty as anyone, wanting to turn in somewhere quick for a bite to eat after working out...but I always remember, my {MTTB} I have food at home waiting for me to cook it, the way I like it. I only dine out now when it becomes a social thing...or it's easier for me to get a quick bite, but I'm still very choosy in selecting my food. That reminds me, an old high school friend that I haven't seen in 30 years commented on Facebook..." *I know you're still a health nut.*" Wow, that made me realize that I've been doing this for a long time.

My last word about Food is to be smart, creative, and appreciative. Take the time to prepare your menu, cook it yourself, and enjoy it. Food is a very important part of putting together your lifelong regimen. Remember, it's a Scientific fact; Vegetables, Fruits, Fish, Poultry, Beef, and Nuts work best with the human body and all can be purchased fresh. In fact, nutritionists in Hospitals, are ordered by the primary physician to prepare a menu for their patients that's the most beneficial for the healing process. For example: Cruciferous vegetables. This reminds me if you're going to start the recovery process of healing your damaged skin, I recommend a Super Green Product. This will deliver healing ingredients where it's most needed, along with a good protein supplement.

CHAPTER 4

~

Sunshine

My method of *"Sunshine Layering"* is the best way of getting the best tan and the health benefits we all need for vitamin D. So, try to expose as much of your body as possible for at least 10-20 minutes a day, preferably between 10:00 am – 11:00 am. Trust me, if you use this method, you will achieve the best tan ever, way better than spray tans or a tanning bed session.

The trick is to be patient, don't rush it by staying out in the sun until you're scorched. The *"fell asleep in the Sun"* is a ridiculous look and dangerous. Scorching your skin when you're young will promote skin cancer later in life.

Some people can spend all their lives in the sun without complications, and some cannot. Nevertheless...I'm here to tell you that every living plant, creature, and human being on Earth needs exposure to the Sun.

Remember, when it comes to tanning, patience is your friend. Slow down, soak up the Sun, little by little and people will comment on how nice your skin looks, instead of, "Wow you got fried" and that's not good. Every time you "Fry" yourself, you've created a potential for manifesting Skin Cancer which could raise its ugly head, later in life, as you grow older. Trust me on this.

I will have to say for the record, I absorbed too much sun being a lifeguard growing up, and glad I'm controlling the exposure.

Just remember, once you've practiced my daily regimen for a while, Sunshine will be the icing on the cake...Brief Moments of Sun Sprinkled down on your skin to help capture your Natural Beauty.

Oh, I know, some might say, that's ridiculous, I will never lay in the sun, and yes, that might be good for some who are very sensitive, even allergic to the sun. But if you live on Planet Earth, you need some Sunshine.

CHAPTER 5

What Supplements Should We Take?

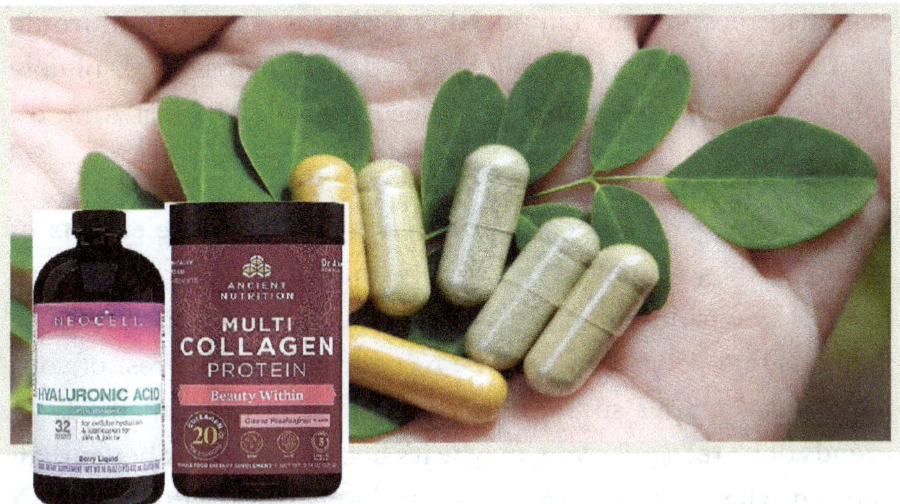

Of course, this will not apply to young adults. It's for those who are a little older and for those who have decided to return to themselves and need a little help. All of us are bombarded with advertisements proclaiming their products provide life-changing events. Yet, after purchasing the product, taking it for months at a time, following the directions explicitly, only to find out later that it was nothing but a waste of time and money, with good advertising. How many times have you done this? You get worked up thinking you've found the answers in a bottle, tube, or box. Only to be disappointed in the quest, time after time...100% of synthetic products will not assimilate into your body for the betterment and may even do harm.

However, let me clue you in for those who may not know, that hyaluronic acid, collagen, and proteins can and will provide the expected results. I recommend **Dr. Axe's Collagen Protein.** There's no taste to it and you can mix it up a couple of times a day in 6-8 ounces of water it dissolves within seconds, or you can add it to a smoothie.

I also recommend Liquid **NEO CELL** as a good **Hyaluronic Acid.** It helps to keep your skin hydrated. I ran across an absolutely good essential supplement we all need, it's called Perfect **Aminos.** (Protein).

I mostly use methods of combining the natural elements of Water, Protein, Minerals, and good whole Foods. Combined with Exercise, Sunshine, organic supplements, and key maintenance methods that will help you to be recognizable for the rest of your life. However, after six months or so of using these methods...if friends don't recognize you, maybe it's because you look better than you did when they last saw you. Maybe it's because they haven't seen the younger-looking-you in a while...

I will admit there are Key Vitamin Supplements you should always take consistently to reap the benefits, help your body maintain overall health, and achieve expected benefits. Start off the day with a few drops of Trace Minerals in an 8oz. a glass of water. Then when you have breakfast take a good multivitamin, and 1000 mg of Vitamin C, since most are eliminated during urination every day. Include good Vitamin D3 liquid drops and B-12 with a Folic Acid supplement. I prefer using a liquid supplement, as your body will absorb much easier, and assimilation is quicker. (Nano)

CHAPTER 6

~

Preferred Skin Regimen Forever

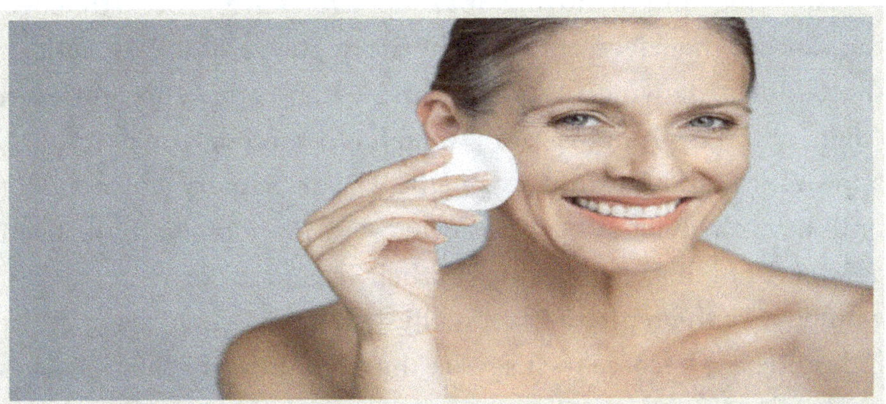

Super Important!

First Let me say this:

You might have seen pictures of women in your family albums noticing how beautiful they were, and probably were not wearing makeup. You can carry on that family beauty by never wearing makeup. Other relatives might say: *"Oh, you look just like your grandmother when she was in her teens."*

I'm not going to apologize for disparaging Hollywood. They've directly or sublimely started the entire beginning of wearing makeup, through their films and Magazines.

It has the largest number of followers on the Planet. But it comes with a price. Wearing makeup and removing it over the years has taken a toll on Hollywood's leading women and even men. Really you ask. Search *"Hollywood's Makeup Before & After"*

Warning it could shock you!

Applying and removing makeup aggressively has stretched the skin on their face and neck horribly. You've probably noticed the tabloids showing them with and without makeup and even "then" and "now" photos. Hollywood has been rough on everyone's appearance, and let's not forget the Plastic Surgery horrors. Not only have their faces been distorted, but their minds have been as well. Thinking that cutting on their face to lift or remove skin, would make them prettier, not really, it only disfigured them. Most hide and have become recluses. It's the price they pay. But that does not have to happen to you.

Hair Dyes and Bleach will take a toll on your hair with constant dying or bleaching. It will begin to thin out, losing the natural ability to absorb the Color desired, having the appearance of Cotton Candy, no matter the color, especially those on prescribed medication, like birth control. Beware....

For Young Women: First, I hope you'll never use makeup to cover, hide, to put a mask over an already perfect face. Be happy with who you are, with what God gave you. Show others that you are who you are, and no one is going to persuade you to do otherwise. Say to yourself: "I am the real thing and what you see, is what you get". "My hair is all-natural, my skin is clean, I am a Natural Beauty from the start and always will be."

For Makeup Users: If you're a current makeup user, I hope someday soon, you'll decide to toss all your makeup and return to yourself. I'm telling you now that the human body is remarkable, and your skin can and will recover to the best it possibly could be. It may not recover as well as if you never wore makeup but will return to the better you.

Some will recover to their younger self. You'll never have to run to put your makeup on to cover the worn-out face, changing into the fake face. You'll be surprised when your boyfriend or husband tells you the things you've wanted to hear, especially those who have been together before you started wearing makeup. Hmmm, maybe the missing romance will return, because I'm here to tell you, wherever I go, I notice women who have returned to themselves, the ones who are not part of the norm any longer. The stress of wearing makeup is over. I want you to say to yourself *"I'm sick of wearing makeup." "It's done nothing for me but wear out the skin on my face." "I will work hard to nourish my body and mind, to recover from all the damage I've done to my natural appearance.*

I WILL RETURN TO MYSELF...

~

Skin Textures

First, I want to say for the record that women of Color have no business wearing makeup. They are the most natural beauties on the Planet. Please, Black women, dark-skinned women should never wear bright colors on their eyelids, and lips. It takes away from their natural features. It distorts their faces making them totally unappealing compared to their own natural self.

Next is the skin on your knees and elbows is of course, not as delicate as the skin under your eyes or your eyelids, right? However, both serve a purpose, as do all areas of skin on your body. The skin on your knees, elbows, hands, and feet serves as a pad for these areas. However, you still will have to care for them as you would for the rest of the skin on your body.

Your eyelids are without a doubt the most delicate, otherwise, you couldn't open and close your eyes so easily, right? The skin on your forehead is still a little different than the skin on your cheeks, chin, and neck, correct? Now that we have understood this, there's a way to cleanse these areas without progressive damage.

This means that from a very young age, it is very easy for one to begin stretching your facial skin. Just like you see guys and girls who wear big earrings with stretched-out ear lobes. Your skin will and does stretch. It is very important to learn this at a very young age. There are methods that will prevent this from happening. It's something you will begin to learn and hopefully, you will master the method before bad habits become routine.

As I stated before, your eyelids are the most fragile, delicate skin on the face. It will stretch very easily. Think about it, it's the first part of your face that reflects aging. If people realized this, they could automatically prevent 10-20 years of aging already. Yet, when removing makeup, or even rubbing their eyes aggressively they unconsciously pull and stretch this thin skin way too much. Every morning you pull on the eyelids by removing the eye rheum, (sleep), rubbing, and using your fingers to do so. Wait!

The more makeup you use or forget to remove at night before going to bed, contributes to morning-eye boogers and clogged pores. Now that you know this, you are the judge of what you're going to put on your eyes and the method you use to take it off. Just remember, you're the one that's pulling, tugging, and pushing on this skin around your eyes, cheeks, and neck, and eventually, it will be stretched out prematurely and could have been prevented. Hopefully, you're not planning to wear makeup on this delicate skin at all. Simply put, if you don't wear makeup, you'll never have to pull or stretch this area on your face.

Return to yourself.... You will not regret it and wonder why you didn't do it a long time ago.

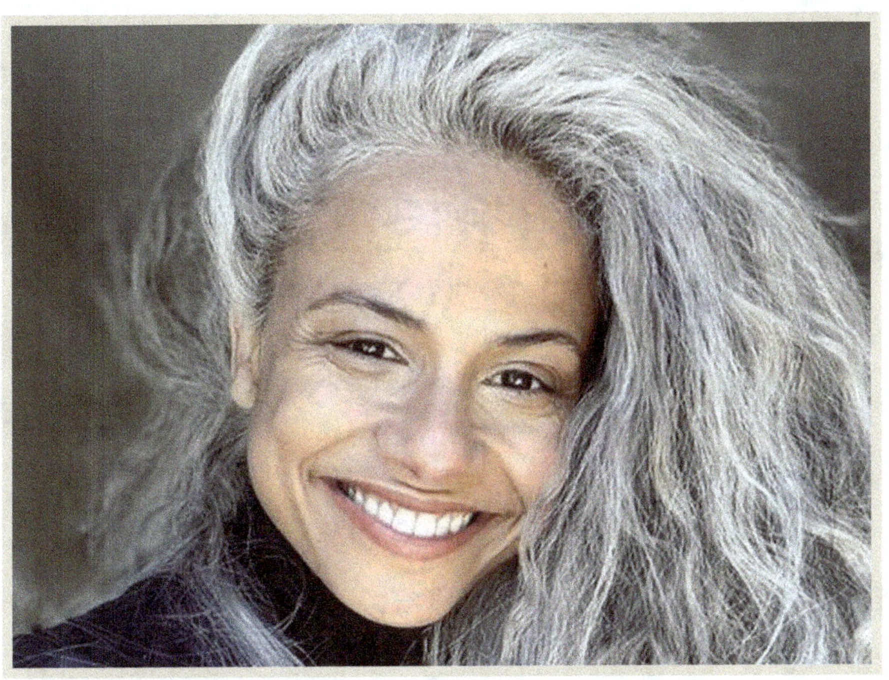

Now you're Perfection without trying...

MY SKIN PRESERVATION AND RECOVERY DIET

~

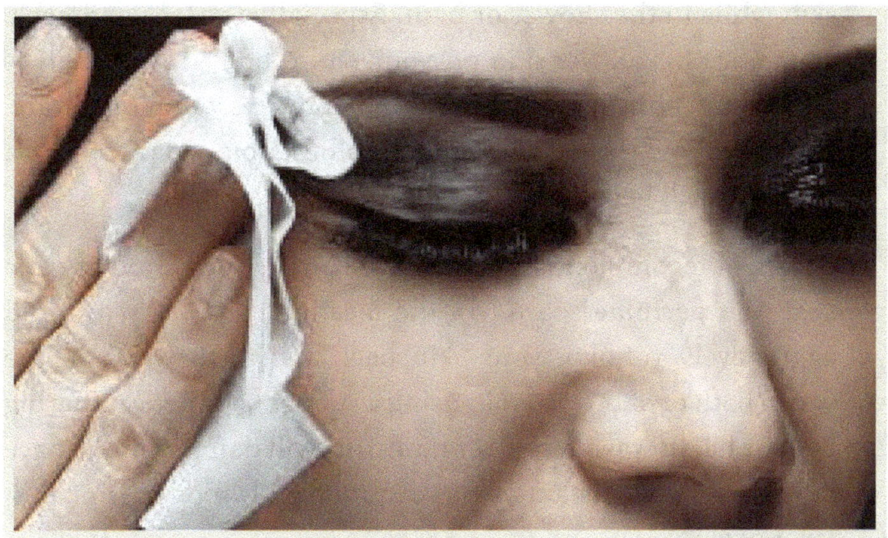

For young women who have never thought about wearing makeup and for those who have decided to stop wearing makeup and continue their life as a Natural Beauty.

First, always remember that your skin will stretch very easily, and over time, you will notice premature aging. So, you'll want to take heed and always be aware of how delicate your skin is.

- **Morning Wake Up** – Your body is warm when you wake in the morning, so always avoid rubbing your eyes aggressively. This takes a huge toll on the skin around the eyes. Simply wait until you get in the shower or splash water on your face to gently remove the sleep. (Rheum)

- **Shower or Bath** – First you'll want to drink at least 8 (1 cup) of water before bathing or showering. Your skin quadruples the chance of stretching when taking a hot/warm bath or shower. So, avoid aggressively using a Wash Rag or just rubbing your skin while in the shower or bath. Especially the face and neck. That goes for all the skin on your entire body. I know this is challenging, but at least this statement makes you more aware. Simply follow these suggestions the best you can, and over a period, it will become second nature to you.

- **Soaps** – I recommend using Goat Milk Soaps or a good organic soap (no perfume soaps) on the face and body. Try to avoid aggressively rubbing your skin back and forth while in the warm bath or shower. Avoid using a sponge, synthetic lathering ball, or harsh wash rag. Over time, this will damage the surface of your skin. A constant abrasive motion will erode the first best layer of skin.

   Washing your face is very important. Always work up a good lather in your hands and gently apply it to the areas intended on your face, using only the pads of your fingers.. Remember, taking a warm or hot shower or bath, your skin will be easy to stretch. Even though you're young and the skin is more resilient, over a period, it will take its toll, so always be aware of the care you give yourself. Easy does it. Now, when rinsing the soap off your face and your body, again, you'll want to use only the pads of your fingers or just the water to gently glide over your face and body, which will gently push out the soap or whatever may be trapped in your pores. Remember, your pores are a vital part of the exhaust system. Never tug on your skin in a warm bath or shower, especially around your eyes. Be ever so gentle.

- **Shampoos** – Try to avoid shampooing your hair every day, this will wash out the natural oils that are good for your scalp and hair. I hope you're a fan of Organic everything, so try to use organic shampoo. Check the ingredients to avoid harsh chemicals and toxins. There are a lot of popular showering products and hairdressings containing carcinogens, so beware and be picky when purchasing your products. When rinsing your hair, continue for several minutes, especially if you have long hair. This is very important. Rinse your hair, then your face, and then the body, then your face again., your face being the last. It may not seem important but if it becomes part of your lifelong regimen, it will make a huge difference in your skin's appearance. A Cold-Water rinse is good. It closes the pores on your body.

Very important, very, very, important.

- **Towel Dry** – Now that you've finished your shower or bath, carefully towel dry by patting and never rubbing. Why? Yes, you're right, because, after the hot/warm bath or shower, your skin is very soft and delicate and will remain easy to Stretch until it's cooled off. If you have the time, lay a towel out on the bed, under a fan, to cool your skin. Do this in your life as often as possible.

- **VERY IMPORTANT**- Rinsing the face one more time. Fill your sink with water, and dump in some ice from your Refrigerator. When it's almost melted completely, begin splashing it on your face and neck. You'll want the water to be very cold, keep doing this for several minutes until it becomes very invigorating, turning your face a pinkish red. Wow! This simple task will provide above and beyond your expectations as a preventative skin regimen for life. It will help your skin recover from bruising and dark circles from the use of makeup. This simple task will preserve your natural beauty. It is your "Fountain of Youth," at your disposal. Very Cool!

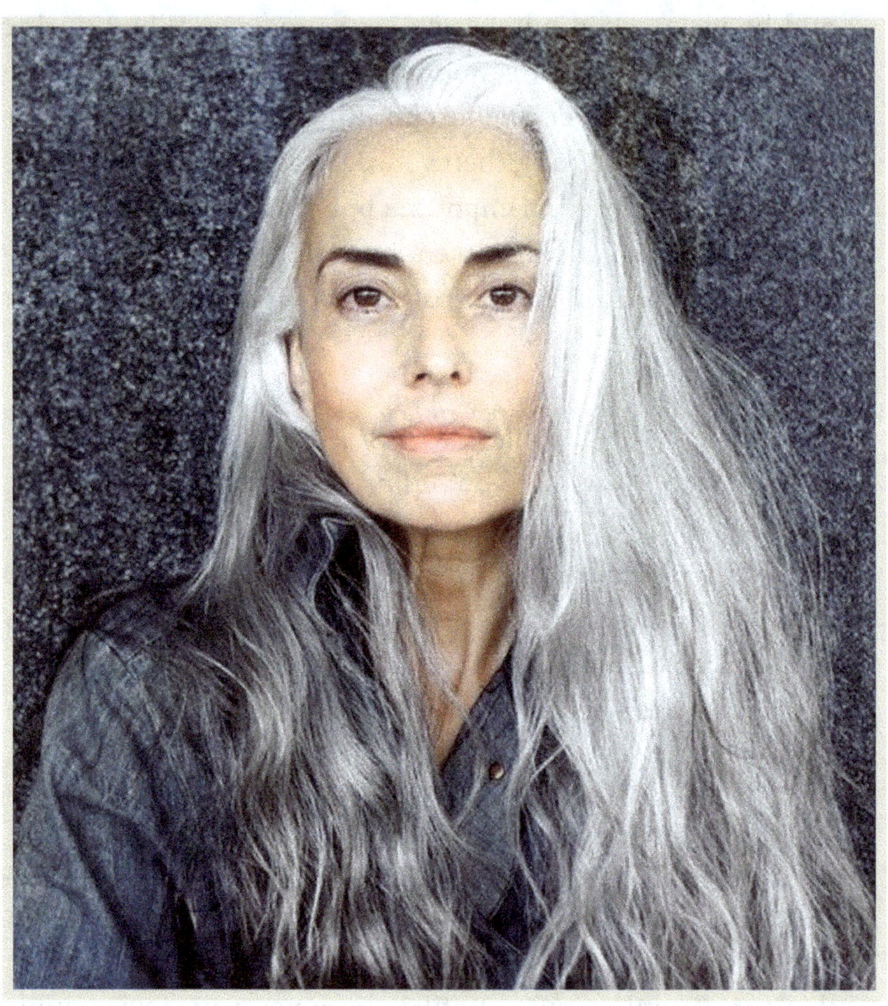

A Natural Beauty

Do you want to be one of those women who will never be worrying about your makeup? Forget about it, and the weight will be lifted off your shoulders. Yes, it may take time to repair the bruises around your eyes as well as dark circles under your eyes, and spots on your face, but through nutrition, a lifelong daily regimen, and exercise, you will return to yourself. A better you. You'll return to the beautiful you, just be consistent and patient and keep on target.

We all age, but why not do it with dignity and without people laughing behind your back? I get sad when I see women trying to look young by using make-up or having plastic surgery. Oh yeah, it turns heads, but in the wrong direction. Months ago, I attended a gathering in Dallas, Texas. I must tell you, the women that turned my head and a lot of others were the women that had natural hair color, long and beautiful, with their eyes shining bright, their skin as radiant as could be for any age. A few had followed my regimen, thanking me for the confidence it gave them, and even their husbands told me it was the best thing that had happened to them since they were in High School, her husband said; *"Her scent had returned, and zapped me back so abruptly, I stared at her while she was talking with friends, realizing I had chosen well for life."*

Sure, they were older, but an older beautiful woman turned more heads and was the talk of the room, looking like natural beauty, so much younger than she was. No more pounds of makeup or dyed hair glued together. You see more Americans than Europeans tend to live their lives behind a mask and plastic surgery. In fact, 100% of women with Plastic Surgery, wear tons of makeup to cover up the surgery scars and imperfections, compounding the unwanted attention, and not in a good way.

Masks: If you want to nourish your face, mix up something natural that will assimilate. They're plenty of suggestions online to choose from. Just search "organic facial creams" These are nutritious food creams for your skin. Always avoid the "dry peeling or clay masks" they do nothing but stretch your skin with every peeling and tugging pull. Don't fall for these sales gimmicks about a peeling-off mask of any kind. I do approve of using a blackhead removal strip just for the nose, rinsing with ice-cold water afterward, but anywhere else will stretch the skin, especially around the eyes.

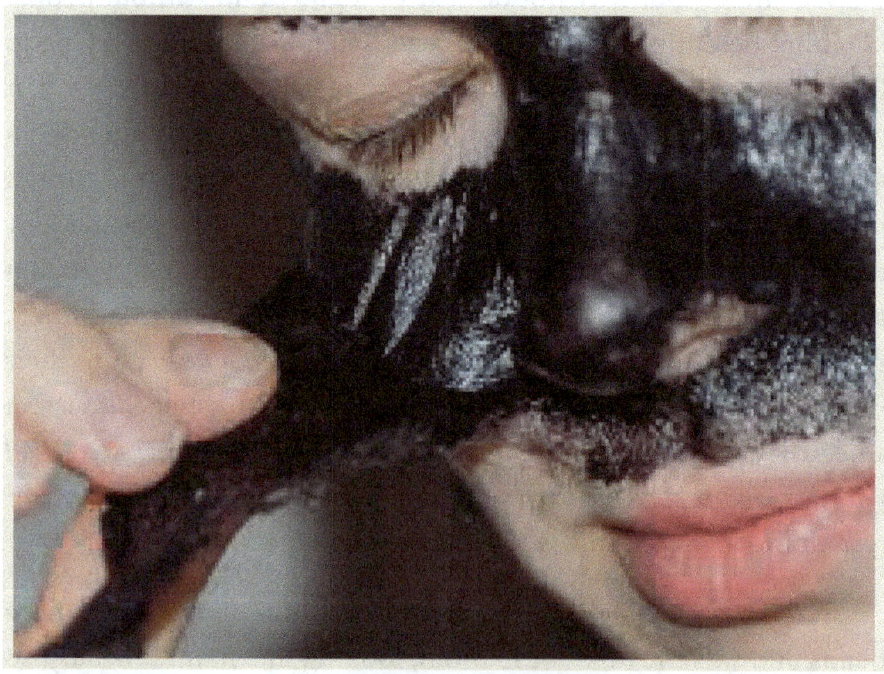

Removing Makeup Every Night Undoubtedly Ages Skin Simply by Stretching and Bruising Over and Over

Helpful Hints:

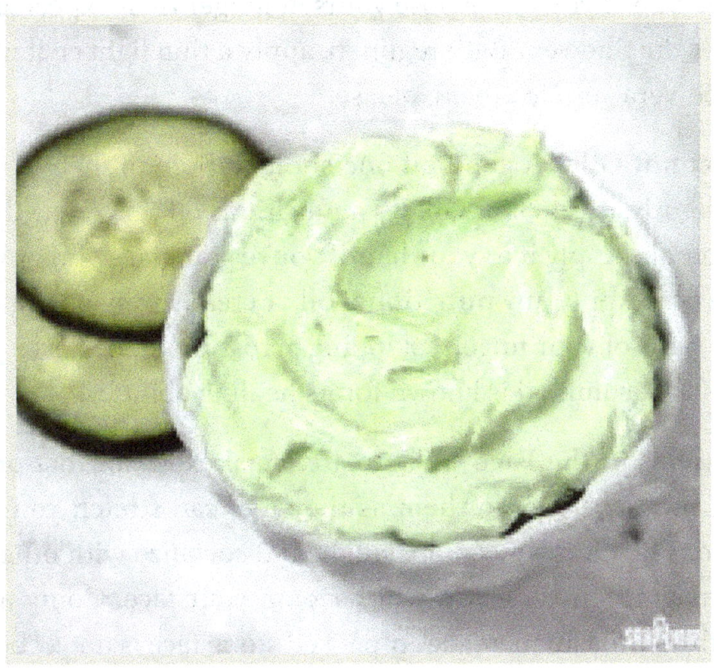

- **Creamy Nutritious Mask** - After using a creamy nutritious mask on your face, rinse with warm water, then finish with ice-cold water. (No peel masks on your facial skin, maybe your nose but that's it.

- **Never Squint** - Never squint or pull down your eyes to see. If you need glasses, see a doctor and get the right prescription to avoid squinting. Absolute worst for the skin around your eyes and forehead.

- **For Men** - When shaving, never stretch your skin with one hand to shave an area hard to see or reach. Over time, this will stretch your skin. You'll end up with more jowl than expected. Try to maintain your normal weight as much as possible.

- **Fun in the Sun** - After playing in the Sun all day, unavoidable right? So, if you did expose yourself longer than expected, then after the Shower / Bath regimen, apply a thin light coat of 100% Aloe Vera gel. No cream, please!

- **Coconut Oil** – A good oil one should apply to their skin ever so lightly, is Coconut Oil. It's a nutritious oil that feeds the skin and hair. Apply it to your hair if you're going to swim or play in the sun. Apply any **nutritional** oil or cream ever so lightly with the balls of your fingers, skipping across the skin. Never pull or push. Coconut oil is known for its healing abilities.

- **Muscles in the Face** – There are facial exercises that one can do, but don't overdo them as they too, can stretch your facial skin. The more you smile, laugh, and socialize with others, the better muscle tone you will have on your face. Going around with a Tardashian, makeup-packed stone face is not a good way to tone your face.

- **Try to stick to your diet of life** every day. Sure, it's challenging, as I mentioned before. But in the long run, you'll have this information for reference and hopefully on your mind. I think day by day, month to month, year to year while referencing this information from time to time, you will unknowingly begin to compose your own regimen. Possibly modifying some and adding more of your own.

The following is a summary for reference.

1. **Waking** – Your face is warm, so don't rub your eyelids, it is thin and very delicate.

2. **Start with water and end with water.** Cleanse your body using your own method but be more aware of your body's skin textures. Use only the pads of your fingers to slightly help to remove soap and debris from your pores. About 1x a month, you can use a volcanic facial Scrub to lightly go over your face and neck areas. Be ever so careful, again using the pads of your fingers to glide over the forehead, nose, chin, around your eyes, and neck. Remember, your skin is warm from the shower, so be gentle with the Face Scrub. You are not trying to scrape off barnacles.

3. **Rinse thoroughly,** especially long hair, rinse with your head tilted back, then forward, then your body, then your face. Always rinse your face last.

4. Rinse with cold water, this is great to help tighten up the pores and close the hair follicles.

5. **Using a towel,** pat or gently slide the towel over your body, never pull or rub aggressively, pushing and tugging, especially if you didn't rinse with cold water. **Please note:** Once you rinse with ice-cold water, it will make a huge impression and

will be embedded in your mind. Repeat the process as much as possible.

6. No **sculpting gels or hairsprays.** (avoid chemicals)

7. **Sunshine** 10-20 minutes of Vitamin D, preferably 11:00 a.m. (Remember, every living thing on the Planet needs Sunshine. I promise you, a 10–20-minute session at a time, will provide you with the most natural glowing skin ever.

8. **NO MAKEUP** Be patient with this process expecting nothing but good results. Your friends will be talking about you, totally envious of the challenge you put yourself through. You can make this happen for yourself, and live stress-free. Very Important

9. **Lip Gloss** to moisten only, not dripping off your lips.

10. A touch of **Fragrance,** but don't bathe in it. You'll want your own scent to come through as well.

11. **Hair** - No Bleach or Color on your hair. Wearing your hair naturally will carry a lot of your natural scent and pheromones. It's what guys remember more than anything when they are away, the scent of a woman's hair. Bleaching or coloring your hair over time will inevitably thin it out and the color will not adhere to the follicles, like it did when you first started.

12. **Organic Oils:** The Only Oils I recommend for the Arms, Legs, Feet, Hands, and Neck are of course, Organic. Choose Any Organic Oil that will assimilate to your body and fit your budget. First, apply it to your hand, and gently glide on to your body. You'll eventually create your own method

from body part to body part, and will inevitably improve the coverage each time you apply. Keep it up!

13. No **creamy-waxy lotions** (Remember don't clog your Exhaust system)

14. **At bedtime**, wash your face with warm soapy water using Organic Goat Milk Soaps or any Organic Soap. Rinse well with warm water then finish with ice cold water. Pat Dry.

Do this in the morning too, especially if you are not going to shower or bathe, at least you can cleanse your face. Then hit the Sun for a short session.

For those who can afford it, have an ice dispenser installed in your bathroom.

MY LAST WORDS ON THE SUBJECT...

~

To me, the word "Diet" means the "way of life". A support plan, necessary for everything you eat, drink, or apply to your body, that will assimilate, allowing you to evolve for the betterment of your body, mind, and soul throughout your entire life. It's the way we were designed. Your body cannot use synthetics of any kind. People say women age faster and more than men their same age. In this book, I explain the primary reasons for premature aging and what you can do to recover. I know it will be challenging at first, to some of you but sooner than you expect, it will become second nature in your daily routines. Some of you will probably modify or create methods that work best for you in your own time. You will begin to create your own lifelong "diet", your own personal healthy regimen. In the end, you will become recognizable to your friends, the real you, a familiar face everyone recognizes. Don't cover that pretty face with makeup. Stand out in your group and be the beautiful young girl you've always been.... with nothing but water and kisses from your mother ever to touch that face.... Remember, as a young girl, you have perfection without trying, and for those who need encouragement to stop wearing makeup and begin the healing process of facial recovery, have faith, and return to yourself. I have faith in you...Victor Christian

NOTES TO REMEMBER...

~

Best Suntan Ever

In 2002 I was in Oxnard, California attending meetings at the main office. During the breaks from the meetings, I would step outside to soak up some rays. No more than 15 minutes at a time. When I returned to Dallas, I noticed that I was getting more attention than usual. Didn't know why, until one person said Wow! That's the best tan ever! Where have you been? What tanning lotion do you use? I guess in those few sessions, the sun not only nourished my skin but left me with an ever-so-layered tan. Ever since then, I knew that method was the one to share. You cannot beat Vitamin D3 from our Sun. Like I said before, every living thing needs sunlight. So the best tan ever is layering the Sunlight 10-20 minutes a day, even in Winter.

Skin Stretching

Natives of African Tribes are known for stretching their ear lobes, and lips with odd ornamental objects. It's without a doubt, Skin will stretch first with gravity, then with influence, as well as gaining weight faster than usual. Like during pregnancy and or bodybuilding. History tells us Trappers would heat animal skins and stretch them on lodge poles to make the skin bigger. The bigger the Skin, the more money they made. **True Story.** I hope this statement will embed itself into your brain to remind you about bathing or showering in warm and hot water

LIST OF THINGS THAT WILL MOST LIKELY CONTRIBUTE TO PREMATURE AGING...

~

1. **Applying and Removing Makeup, without a doubt is the primary reason for premature aging for men and women. A costly mistake for those who want to look young for as long as they possibly can.**

2. **Smoking** – Causes wrinkles around the lips, mouth, and chin, from the constant movement of drawing the smoke and drying out the pigment in your skin. Plus, smoking without a doubt is a detriment to your body, inside and out. Makes your breath smell bad too. Don't smoke.

3. **Alcohol** – drinking wreaks havoc on your skin and body. It contributes to restricting moisture in the skin and restricts blood flow.

4. **Poor Nutritious Diet- Undoubtedly promotes skin problems.**

5. **Weight Gain** – If you become overweight, to the point where your face, arms, and legs get fat, then you get older and lose a lot of weight, your skin will be loose, wrinkled, and crepey.

6. **Lack of Sleep** – Every human needs adequate sleep to maintain good health and vitality.

7. **Exercise** is a must for every human. Stimulates the cells necessary for maintaining a young vibrant appearance.

8. **Hot shower** - Never begin rubbing, pulling, or tugging on your skin aggressively, while taking a warm or hot shower.

9. **Optimum Hydration** Stay hydrated, supplementing your water with electrolytes and trace minerals.

www.ingramcontent.com/pod-product-compliance
Lightning Source LLC
Chambersburg PA
CBHW050836260726
48660CB00006B/2272